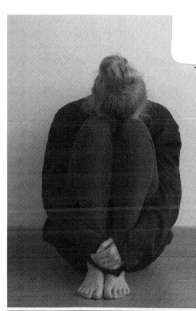

VASCULAR DEMENTIA

Activities for the Family Caregiver
HOW TO ENGAGE, HOW TO LIVE

Endorsed by

National Council of
Certified Dementia Practitioners

Scott Silknitter, Robert D. Brennan
and Alisa Tagg

Disclaimer

This book is for informational purposes only and is not intended as medical advice, diagnosis, or treatment. Always seek advice from a qualified physician about medical concerns, and do not disregard medical advice because of something you read within this book. This book does not replace the need for diagnostic evaluation, ongoing physician care, and professional assessment of treatments. Every effort has been made to make this book as complete and helpful as possible. It is important, however, for this book to be used as a resource and idea-generating guide and not as an ultimate source for plan of care.

ISBN # 978-1-943285-18-1

Published by
R.O.S. Therapy Systems, L.L.C.
Greensboro, NC
888-352-9788
www.ROSTherapySystems.com

Activities for the Family Caregiver—Vascular Dementia

There are many causes for dementia. Vascular dementia is considered by many to be one of the top three causes.

No matter the cause, dementia takes a toll on everyone involved. It certainly did for our family and that is why this book and our company were born. A simple backyard project during my father's 25-year battle with Parkinson's and dementia has turned into a company with a simple mission to help all families caring for a loved one.

This book was written as a basic guide to help family caregivers engage their loved one and make life a little more enjoyable. Whether it is accomplishing activities of daily living, such as bathing, or engaging in a conversation to prevent boredom and wandering, our goal is to make things a little easier and less stressful by providing common sense suggestions and tools to engage your loved one.

With the assistance of Robert D. Brennan, RN, NHA, MS, CDP, and Alisa Tagg, BA, ACC/EDU, AC-BC, CDP, who have been working in long-term care for a combination of 60 years, we have written this book full of "How To's" and "Why's" to help you.

We hope you find this book useful, and we encourage you to have other family members and caregivers read this. This is the first step to consistency with approaches, verbal cues, physical assistance, and modifications that produce positive results for your loved one.

From our family of caregivers to yours, please remember that you are not alone, and to never give up.

Scott Silknitter

Table of Contents

Family Members and Caregivers
that have read this book:

_____

_____

_____

_____

_____

_____

_____

_____

_____

_____

_____

_____

Chapter 1

Vascular Dementia Overview

Vascular dementia, also known as Vascular Cognitive Impairment (VCI), is a disease resulting in symptoms of dementia as well as other physical and psychological challenges.

Vascular dementia occurs after injury to the blood vessels of the brain. Vascular dementia will affect people in numerous and different ways depending on the location of these blood vessels within the brain.

A review from *Activities 101 for the Family Caregiver—Vascular Dementia*: Vascular dementia is a decline in thinking skills caused by conditions that block or reduce blood flow to various regions of the brain, depriving brain cells of vital oxygen and nutrients. In vascular dementia, changes in thinking skills sometimes occur suddenly following a stroke that blocks major blood vessels in the brain. Thinking difficulties may also begin as mild changes that can worsen gradually as a result of multiple minor strokes or other conditions that affect smaller blood vessels, leading to cumulative damage.

The impact of vascular conditions on thinking skills varies widely, depending on the severity of the blood vessel damage and the part of the brain it affects. Memory loss may or may not be a significant symptom depending on the specific brain areas where blood flow is reduced. Vascular damage that starts in brain areas that play a key role in storing or retrieving information may cause memory loss that looks very much like Alzheimer's disease.

Symptoms due to vascular dementia may be most obvious when they happen soon after a major stroke.

Any condition that damages blood vessels throughout your loved one's body may have caused brain changes linked to vascular

dementia. Additional factors are the same
ones that raise your risk for heart problems,
stroke, and other diseases that affect blood
vessels. The following strategies may reduce
your risk including:

- Don't smoke.
- Keep your blood pressure, cholesterol,
  and blood sugar within recommended
  limits.
- Eat a healthy, balanced diet.
- Exercise.
- Maintain a healthy weight.
- Limit alcohol consumption.

People who suffer from vascular dementia can
benefit greatly from participation in daily
activities. Some benefits from engaging in
activities are:

- Enjoy happier daily life.
- Increase feelings of self-worth.
- Enhance and maintain general health.

- Maintain memory.
- Enhance and maintain communication skills.
- Improve and increase personal relationships.
- Preserve family history.
- Strengthen and maintain muscles.
- Reduce muscle and joint pain.
- Increase and maintain flexibility.
- Reduce nervous tension.
- Decrease pacing and restlessness.
- Decrease repetitive behaviors.
- Decrease wandering.
- Increase nighttime sleep.

Risk factors for vascular dementia are similar to those resulting in a cerebrovascular stroke. They include:

- Increased age
- High blood pressure

- Diabetes
- High cholesterol
- Atrial fibrillation
- History of heart attack/stroke
- Smoking

Symptoms of vascular dementia can, as with a stroke, occur suddenly or over a period of time. The symptoms can also progress or subside at a later time.

Signs and Symptoms

Emotional and Mental

- Slowed thinking
  - Taking longer to process what is said and answering questions.
- Confusion which may get worse at night
  - This is called "sun-downing." Your loved one becomes easily agitated or confused when the sun goes down.

- Loss of social skills
  - Inability to express oneself or carry a conversation.
- Memory problems
  - Unable to remember what they ate for breakfast or if they ate at all.
- General forgetfulness
  - Unable to remember people including family members or remembering how items work.

Physical

- Dizziness
- Leg or arm weakness
- Balance problems
- Tremors
- Loss of bladder or bowel control
- Slurred speech since Sept'21

Behavioral

- Language problems
  - Using the wrong words. Often called "word salad."

- Getting lost in familiar surroundings
  - Forgetful of where they need to go or forgetting how to get home.
- Difficulty planning, organizing, following instructions
  - Unable to follow directions because when the directions are given they can't remember what was said.
- Reduced ability to function in daily life
  - Unable to keep up with activities of daily living, such as bathing self, brushing teeth, going to the bathroom, or eating properly.

Other types of vascular dementia include:

Multi-Infarct Dementia

Multi-infarct dementia occurs when many small strokes damage the brain cells. One side of the brain may be affected more than the other. Damage may only affect a certain area of the brain and symptoms will vary depending on the area affected.

If these small strokes occur on both sides of the brain, there is a higher chance of vascular dementia symptoms developing. In some instances, a single stroke can result in significant dementia (known as single-infarct dementia).

Subcortical Vascular Dementia (Binswanger's Disease):

This is a rare form of vascular dementia that results from microscopic damage to small blood vessels and nerve fibers of the brain's white matter.

A characteristic symptom of Binswanger's disease is known as "psychomotor slowness." This can be observed when an individual is taking a substantial amount of time to think of a letter and then write it down.

Symptoms/problems are associated with this form of vascular dementia:

- Short-term memory
- Organization

- Mood
- Attention
- Decision making
- Appropriate behavior

Some examples could be that your loved one forgets what the keys are used for or puts the cereal in the fridge and the milk in the cupboard.

In addition, there may be urinary incontinence, trouble walking, clumsiness, and lack of facial expression.

The level of symptoms and dementia present is directly related to the extent of the damage that has occurred.

CADASIL

Cerebral Autosomal Dominant Arteriopathy with Subcortical Infarcts and Leukoencephalopathy (CADASIL) was formerly known as hereditary multi-infarct dementia.

This is an inherited (genetic) form of cardiovascular disease resulting in the walls of blood vessels (small and medium in size) thickening and reducing the necessary blood flow to the brain. Most individuals with CADASIL have a family history of the disorder.

This form of vascular dementia is associated with:

- Multi-infarct dementia
- Stroke
- Migraine with auras
- Mood disorders

Age of onset is usually between the age of 20 and 40. Symptoms and disease onset vary widely, typically appearing in the mid-30s. Some individuals may not show signs of the disease until later in life.

Symptoms usually progress slowly. By age 65, the majority of persons with CADASIL have

cognitive problems and dementia. Some
will become physically dependent due to
multiple strokes.

Examples of this include:

- An inability to properly
  communicate needs, such as
  going to the bathroom.

- An increase in wandering
  without purpose.

- Becoming more forgetful of
  tasks at hand.

- An inability to sleep at night.

Symptoms will develop according to the
amount of vessels destroyed from the disease
process. Your loved one may also show several
of the symptoms you would see with
Alzheimer's or other forms of dementia.

Chapter 2

Activities, Their Benefits, and Help You Bring In

Vascular dementia may or may not affect your loved one's personality, but it does affect their ability to interpret and deal with their surroundings as they did in the past.

Most people with vascular dementia are able to participate in some leisure and pleasurable activities. Everyone is unique, including your loved one; because of this, they will respond to activities or prompts according to their levels of mental abilities, physical abilities, and personal interests.

Vascular dementia is a physical condition, which results in symptoms of dementia—it is not a mental illness. However, individuals may suffer from both.

"Activities" and "Activities of Daily Living" (ADLs) are critical parts of caring for a loved one at home. They both require knowledge of your loved one's habits, preferences, abilities, and routines. That is the foundation for engaging your loved one. Caregivers need to have the ability to communicate with and execute a planned activity with your loved one.

All activities should be planned to offer the best opportunity to enhance your loved one's sense of well-being and reduce your stress. However, "Life happens." Unplanned events, big or small, happen to everyone, and can disrupt the day, the week, or the month. Having the flexibility to adjust to what is happening with your loved one because "Life happened" that day is vital.

Activities should promote and enhance your loved one's physical, cognitive, and emotional health. In this book, we will focus on leisure activities and the activities of daily living with common sense approaches. We will offer suggestions and tips on the "How To's" of getting your loved one engaged, dressed, and fed.

Our goals with this book are to:

1. Provide family caregivers the knowledge and tools to allow them to engage their loved one so that both can enjoy the benefits of activities.

2. Offer a starting point that will provide continuity of approach regarding care, communication, and information-gathering to minimize changes and acclimation time if your loved one does have to move from home to an institutional setting.

Everyone needs to be on the same page. If you choose to use the services of a home care agency while caring for your loved one at home, please ask if they have a Home Care Certified professional on staff, and make sure that the caregiver you choose has received basic training on Leisure Activities and Activities of Daily Living. This will assist with continuity of approach, communication, and planning activities/care that will benefit both you and your loved one.

Our goal is to help you deliver meaningful programs of interest to your loved one that focus on physical, social, spiritual, cognitive, and recreational activities. Everyone involved in the care for your loved one should be "on the same page" to minimize changes and challenges that your loved one will face.

The importance of understanding your family dynamics and the importance of the role each and every individual plays in the care of your loved one is critical. As the dementia progresses, roles will evolve, and everyone needs to understand that this is a process.

If family or friends offer help, accept it with a caveat. Accept the help with their commitment to use the same techniques, strategies, and communication skills that the entire "team" uses.

Being a primary caregiver is a 24/7 job. Without help, you are always on call and run the risk of becoming physically and mentally exhausted.

When you do bring in help, make sure all of your loved one's caregivers (full-time, part-time, family, and/or friends) use the same approach for activities and interaction that you do. With a common approach, there are significantly less opportunities to disrupt routines and make unsettling changes that affect you and your loved one long after the help has left.

A common approach is key. Demand it!

The Four Pillars of Activities

There are four areas that you should focus
on for engaging your loved one in any
type of activity. We call them the Four Pillars
of Activities.

First Pillar of Activities: Know your Loved One—Information Gathering and Assessment

Have a Personal History Form completed.
Know them—who they are, who they were,
and what their functional abilities are today.
Make sure all caregivers know this as well.

Second Pillar of Activities: Communicating and Motivating for Success

Communication is key. Each caregiver
must know how to effectively communicate
with your loved one and be consistent
with techniques.

Third Pillar of Activities: Customary Routines and Preferences

As best as possible, maintain a routine and daily plan based on your loved one's needs and preferences.

Fourth Pillar of Activities: Planning and Executing Activities

Based on all of the information you have gathered about your loved one, you have the opportunity to offer engaging activities that are appropriate and meet your loved one's personal preferences.

The Benefits of Activities with a Standard Approach

Caregiver Benefits of Standard Approach to Activities

Planned and well-executed activities result in less stress for the caregiver as well as less stress for your loved one. Whether the activity involves playing a game or bathing, a standard approach where as many details as possible are pre-planned can make a significant, positive difference for everyone.

Social Benefits of Activities

Activities offer the opportunity for increased social interaction between family members, friends, caregivers, and the one being cared for. Activities create positive experiences and memories for everyone.

Behavioral Benefits of Activities

Well-planned and well-executed activities of any type can reduce challenging behaviors that sometimes arise when caring for someone with dementia.

Self-Esteem Benefits of Activities

Leisure activities offered at the right skill level provide your loved one with an opportunity for success. This is also true with Activities of

Daily Living, such as dressing. Success during activities improves how your loved one feels about themselves.

Sleep Benefits of Activities

As part of a daily routine, activities can improve sleeping at night. If a loved one is inactive all day, it is likely they will nap periodically. Napping can interrupt good sleep patterns at night.

sleeps too much [handwritten marginal note]

Chapter 3

First Pillar of Activities:
Know Your Loved One—
Information Gathering
and Assessment

Know your loved one—The First Pillar of Activities.

What does your loved one enjoy doing?

What do you need to provide care?

Is your loved one capable of doing something independently?

This may vary greatly from what they could do prior to the onset of vascular dementia and may change frequently. ✗

Caregivers

Who is your loved one the most comfortable with when needing care? Female/male, a specific caregiver?

Caregivers will spend considerable time
one-to-one with your loved one, and
it is important that your loved one
feel comfortable.

Illnesses and Limitations

Balance
Weakness
Catheters
Anemia
Swallow

What physical illness or limitations does your
loved one have? What type of modifications
are needed, if any? These, in addition to your
loved one's personal history information, are
just as important to know so that all caregivers
can provide the highest level of care.

Details matter. Gather as much information as
you can for yourself and all caregivers who
may help your loved one.

Basic knowledge about your loved one is
essential. The little things matter.

There are two important items that you
should understand.

First, any form that is used to gather your loved one's personal history should be a living document. It needs constant updating as the dementia progresses. With dementia, what works today may not work tomorrow or may not work five minutes from now!

Second, you and your loved one may have been very private people. Having dementia will change this. Gathering information and sharing information with other caregivers is critical. Your loved one's past pleasures, likes, and activities will become cornerstones of the communication process for everyone.

It is important that before you begin providing personal care, you first need to recognize various personal attributes and abilities of your loved one and yourself. The more you know about your loved one's lifestyle, likes, and dislikes, the easier providing for their personal and leisure needs will be.

If there is something that happened years ago that you consider embarrassing or private, and you choose not to share the information, please note that one way or another, it will come out.

Whatever it was that you think is difficult to share, caregivers and family members that offer assistance are not there to judge you or your loved one on something that happened years or even decades ago. They are there to help you in your current moment of need. Information is vital to the communication process and allows all caregivers the opportunity to turn a "bad" day into a "good" day through proper communication techniques.

As the primary caregiver, you may already know most of the answers, but this is a good and necessary exercise for you, other family members, and caregivers to execute. We suggest everyone fill out the R.O.S. Personal History Form which comes at the end of this book and is also available for download at www.StartSomeJoy.com. As a starting point, you, the primary caregiver, are most likely able to provide the following basic information:

Basic Information

- Name, preferred name to be called, age, and date of birth

Background Information

- Place of birth, cultural/ethnic background, marital status, children (how many, and their names), religion/church, military service/employment, education level, and primary language spoken

Medical and Dietary/Nutritional Information

- Any formal diagnosis, allergies, and food regimen/diets

Habits

- Drinking/alcohol, smoking, exercise, and other things that are a daily habit *Must brush teeth —*

Physical Status

- Abilities/limitations, visual aids, hearing deficits, speech, communication, hand dominance, and mobility/gait

Mental Status

- Alertness, cognitive abilities/limitations, orientation to family, time, place, person, routine, etc.

Social Status

- One-on-one interaction, being visited, communicating with others through written word or phone calls, other means *email*

Emotional Status

- Level of contentment, outgoing/withdrawn, extroverted/introverted, dependent/independent

Leisure Status

- Past, present, and possible future interests

Vision Status

- Any impairment they may have

Functional Levels

In addition to the Personal History, you also need to look at your loved one's functional level. When planning meaningful activities based on individual interests, you have to consider your loved one's functional abilities. Focus on what they *can do* and set them up for success based on what they are able to accomplish. There are several definitions of functional levels. For the purposes of this topic, we will address the following four functioning levels:

Level 1

Your loved one has good social skills. They are able to communicate. They are alert and oriented to person, place, and time, and they have a long attention span.

Level 2

Your loved one has less social skills, and their verbal skills may be impaired as well. Your loved one may have some behavior symptoms. They may need something to do, and they may have an increased energy level, but they have a shorter attention span.

Level 3

Your loved one has less social skills. Their verbal skills are even more impaired than they were at Level 2. They are also easily distracted. Your loved one may have some visual/spatial perception and balance concerns, and they need maximum assistance with their care.

Level 4

Your loved one has a low energy level, nonverbal communication skills, and they rarely initiate contact with others, however, they may respond if given time and cues.

With your loved one's personal history and functional level information, you and every caregiver have the greatest opportunity to provide person-appropriate activities for your loved one.

Chapter 4

Second Pillar of Activities: Communicating and Motivating for Success

Communicating and motivating is the Second Pillar for success in engaging in an activity with your loved one. Because communication and approaches will become difficult early in vascular dementia, recognizing your loved one's ability to understand what is being said is significant to your success in caregiving.

The key to effective communication is the ability to listen attentively with your ears and eyes and using the knowledge of your loved one's lifestyle and habits.

Remember, being logical and/or arguing with your loved one won't work, and in fact could make the situation worse.

Your loved one may not be able to process their environment or what they are doing at any given moment, but they are constantly reading and reacting to your facial expressions, tone of voice, and body language.

Effective Communication Techniques

- Be patient and calm. Use a warm, gentle tone of voice.

- Talk to them like an adult.

- Always smile. Look directly at your loved one.

- Speak slowly with words they know. Use short, simple sentences. Repeat as you need to.

- Give one instruction at a time. Repeat as often as needed.

- Gently touch or hold your loved one's hand while talking, if tolerated.

- Complete one step at a time.

- When they finish one step, go to the next.

- Repeat steps as needed.

- When your loved one is trying to communicate, stop what you are doing, and really listen to what they are *trying* to tell you.

- Give time for your loved one to do or answer.

- Turn questions into statements:

  Instead of, "Do you have to go to the bathroom?" Change to, "The bathroom is right here."

  Instead of, "Would you like a sandwich?" Change to, "Your favorite sandwich is ready."

  Instead of, "Do you want to watch TV?" Change to, "Look, your favorite show is on."

  The point of this is that decision making and judgment are often impaired. Limiting options makes choosing easier. You want to guide your loved one.

Being a Detective

As your loved one's dementia progresses, there will be many days that you will not know what kind of day it will be until after it has started. If there is an issue, the starting point in your process is communicating to figure out what they are telling you.

Validation *vs. Reality orientation*

In 1963, after years of working with oriented, healthy elderly in community centers, Naomi Feil, the developer of Validation Therapy techniques, began working with people over the age of 80 who were disoriented. Her initial goals were to help these people face reality and relate to each other in a group. In 1966, she concluded that helping them to face reality is unrealistic. Each person was trapped in a world of fantasy. Exploring feelings and reminiscing encouraged group members to respond better to each. Music stimulated group cohesion and feelings of well-being.

Mrs. Feil said, "I abandoned the goal of reality orientation when I found group members withdrew, or became increasingly hostile, whenever I tried to orient them to an intolerable present reality."

To validate is to acknowledge the feelings of a person. To validate is to say that their feelings are true. Denying feelings invalidates the individual. Validation uses empathy to tune into the inner reality of the disoriented old-old. Empathy, or walking in the shoes of the other, builds trust. Trust brings safety. Safety brings strength. Strength renews feelings of worth. Worth reduces stress. With empathy, the Validation worker picks up their clues and helps put their feelings into words. This validates them and restores dignity.

The goals of validation are:

- Restore self-worth
- Reduce stress
- Justify living

- Work towards resolving unfinished conflicts from the past
- Reduce the need for chemical and physical restraints
- Increase verbal and nonverbal communication
- Prevent withdrawal inward to vegetation
- Improve gait and physical well-being

Mrs. Feil is a pioneer, and we encourage every caregiver to use validation instead of reality orientation. Here is an example: Your 72-year-old father has vascular dementia that has progressed significantly. One morning he wakes up yelling for Sue. Sue was your mother. Your parents had been married for fifty years, and your mother passed away five years ago.

Your father has woken up looking for his wife and wondering where she is. Actually he has been yelling throughout the house looking for her.

For you, this has been a particularly challenging morning as you have only had a couple of hours of uninterrupted sleep as one of your kids was up throughout the night vomiting because of the flu.

So, you are exhausted, and your father is yelling through the house for his wife who has died. You have a choice to make.

1. You can either look at him and say, "Dad, Mom is not here. She died a few years ago, don't you remember?" or

2. You can look at your father and say, "Dad, Mom is not here. She had to run an errand for me because the kids are sick. I want to make her favorite breakfast for helping me this morning. Please come help me, and tell me how she likes her eggs."

The choice of validation or reality orientation is up to you. If you choose validation, make sure that every caregiver or family member who helps with your loved one knows this. They must use it as well to avoid potential conflicts.

There are simple strategies to communicating with your loved one after you have covered the basics of verbal, nonverbal, and validation. No matter how tired or how upset you may be at your situation, in the heat of the moment, please remember to:

Be Calm

Always approach your loved one in a relaxed and calm demeanor. Your mood will be mirrored by your loved one. Smiles are contagious.

Be Flexible

There is no right or wrong way of completing a task. Offer praise and encouragement for the effort your loved one puts into a task. If you see your loved one becoming overwhelmed or frustrated, stop the task, and re-approach at another time.

Be Nonresistive

Don't force tasks on your loved one. Adults do not want to be told, "No!" or told what to do. The power of suggestion goes a long way, and you get more with an ounce of sugar than you do a pound of vinegar.

Be Guiding, but Not Controlling

Always use a soft, gentle approach, and remember your tone of voice. Your facial expressions must match the words you are saying.

Things to Remember

- Just because your loved one may shake their head yes or no during a discussion, does not always mean your loved one understands or even hears what you or another caregiver is saying. Your loved one may not want to admit they have not understood or heard you.

- Behavior can either enhance and encourage communication or shut it down altogether. You need to assess your listening style and be able to assess the listening styles of the other caregivers and family members working with your loved one.

- It's imperative that all caregivers are on the same page and aware of behaviors, triggers, routines, interventions, and daily tasks of your loved one. They need to use communication techniques that provide an open, nonthreatening environment for your loved one.

Chapter 5

Third Pillar of Activities: Customary Routines and Preferences

Customary routines and preferences is the Third Pillar in an activities program. With vascular dementia, customary daily living and preferences may change when least expected.

Caregiving is a daily routine. The goal is to gain from your loved one's perspective how important certain aspects of care/activity are of interest to them as an individual. This will be difficult. As their abilities to communicate and engage in their environment decreases, your loved one's past interests may no longer be pertinent.

Be aware and be prepared for the potential disruption to *your* personal daily routine. When caring for your loved one at home, this can become very wearing for you.

Daily Customary Routine

Your loved one has distinct lifestyle preferences and routines. They should be preserved to the greatest extent possible with vascular dementia. All reasonable accommodation should be made to maintain their lifestyle preferences.

Always understand, know, and remember that longtime preferences may change as a result of the vascular dementia.

Even though changes to lifelong preferences may occur, your loved one's lifestyle preferences and routine still need to be accommodated as much as possible. When a person feels like their control has been removed and that their preferences are not respected as an individual, it can be demoralizing.

Activity Preferences

Activities are a way for individuals to establish meaning in their lives. A lack of opportunity to engage in meaningful and enjoyable activities can result in boredom, depression, and behavioral disturbances.

Here are some activity suggestions that can be helpful. It is always good when the caregiver utilizes whatever is around the house.

If your loved one likes automobiles:

- Share the history of when the car was first built.
- Attend a local car show.
- Collect and display miniature cars.
- Go for a ride, talk about the sites along the way.
- Look through pictures of cars.
- Reminisce about driving experiences.
- Go online to do research on cars.

**There are more examples of activities in Chapter 7.

Individuals vary in the activities they prefer, reflecting unique personalities, past interests, perceived environmental constraints, religious, and cultural background, and changing physical and mental abilities. Remember, these can and will change with vascular dementia. That is why we use the Personal History Form as a starting point and then engage with Lesson Plans, which are covered in the following chapter. Both of these are intended to be living documents for all caregivers to use, update, and learn from.

Chapter 6

Fourth Pillar of Activities:
Planning and Executing Activities

Planning and executing is the Fourth Pillar
of Activities. With the knowledge of your
loved one's history, functional level, which
communication techniques to use, and
the daily routine, we now look at planning
activities in which your loved one can
be successful.

The Lesson Plan

The Lesson Plan template is a guideline for an
activity. Your loved one's abilities and
responses may be different from one day to
the next, and this will dictate how you modify
an activity to meet their individual needs and
abilities. The Lesson Plan is an ever-changing
document. It is meant to be written on to note
any changes needed so the next person

working with your loved one can follow your modifications in hopes of recreating a positive experience.

Items in the Lesson Plan

Date

Document the date the program is used.

Program Name

You can rename the program if you or your loved one prefer.

Objective of Activity

Our goal is to provide meaningful activities. People have a need to be productive, and they want to engage in something with a purpose. List the objectives of the program.

Materials

The list of suggested materials to use with this program.

Prerequisite Skills

The skills your loved one needs to participate in this program.

Activity Outline

Step-by-step instructions to complete this program.

Evaluation

When you or a family member are conducting an activity with your loved one, documenting results and responses are critical to improve activity programs for your loved one. Items to document:

- Verbal cues, physical assistance or modifications you make to activity.

- Your loved one's response to this program, such as:

    o They actively participated and enjoyed

    o They sat with their arms crossed and head turned away

- Was the activity successful at distracting or eliminating a negative behavior?

A blank template is included on the next page to give you an example of what a Lesson Plan looks like.

Lesson Plan Blank Example

Date	Program Name

Objective of Activity

Materials

Prerequisite Skills

Activity Outline

Evaluation

Chapter 7

Leisure Activity Categories, Types, and Tips

Activity Categories

Activities are generally broken down into three different categories: Maintenance Activities, Supportive Activities, and Empowering Activities.

Maintenance Activities

Maintenance activities are traditional activities that help your loved one to maintain physical, cognitive, social, spiritual, and emotional health. Examples include:

- Using manipulative games, such as those in the R.O.S. Legacy System

- Craft and art activities

- Attending church services

- Working trivia and crossword puzzles like the *How Much Do You Know About* puzzles
- Going on a walk

Supportive Activities

Supportive activities are for loved ones who have a lower tolerance for traditional activities. These types of activities provide a comfortable environment while providing stimulation or solace. Examples include:

- Listening to and singing music
- Hand massages
- Relaxation activities
    - Aromatherapy
    - Meditation
    - Bird-watching

Empowering Activities

Empowering activities help your loved one attain self-respect by receiving opportunities

for self-expression and responsibility.
Examples include:

- Cooking
- Making memory boxes *pictures*
- Folding laundry ✓

Activity Types

Once you have chosen an activity from a category that will suit your loved one's need, you must choose an activity type that will interest them. There are several types of activities to choose from. Below are some examples:

Card Games

Card games are some of the easier games to play. Adjusting the rules as needed to ensure positive self-esteem is okay, too.

*NOTE: Many groups will make the blanket suggestion to "play cards." You must identify your loved one's strengths and weaknesses,

51

and adjust the game played accordingly. Set your loved one up for success, not failure.

- Play Go Fish.

- Play memory matching with pictures of family members. Print pictures that are stored on a computer, and turn them into cards.

- Uno—utilize the Uno cards with color matching or number matching. It is easier to remove the word-written cards. This is fun to do.

Clothing and Laundry *No to almost all*

From the time we were younger, clothing has always been a part of the routine. It is important to encourage your loved one to do as much as possible.

- Practice buttoning shirts or blouses.

- Check garments for loose buttons and learn how to sew them on.

- ✓ Fold handkerchiefs.

- Go to a fashion show.

- Shopping—it may be less confusing to look at catalogs or online.

- Hand wash underwear or socks.

- Hang clothes on a hanger.

- Iron clothes—caregiver will need to monitor.

- Organize shoes in the closet.

- Polish shoes.

- Put clothing away in drawers.

- Put dirty clothing into hamper.

- Tie shoelaces.

Exercise

Exercise is very important. Regular movement helps keep muscles toned and bowel movements regular. Here are some suggestions:

- Pat a balloon back and forth.

Nerf ✓

- Bounce or play catch with a ball (you can select ball size and weight dependent on level).

- Dance.

✓ Lift light "weights" (soup cans, 1 lb. weights, or even unbreakable plastic containers like small water bottles).

- Walk outside (weather dependent) or through an indoor mall.

- Utilize rubber stretch bands for movement.

- Find exercise videos online to work out with. There are seated level videos available.

✓ **Family and Photos**

Family photos are a great way for reminiscing and memory improvement. People with memory loss usually do better at remembering names of cousins and schoolmates in old childhood photos.

- Buy a special frame or decorate one to hold a favorite family photo.
- Have a family group photo taken.
- Keep a journal of family experiences your loved one remembers.
- Share a family story with a relative, perhaps a child, and answer questions.
- Sort through family photos—document names, places, and dates. *and prof.*
- Talk about family experiences—write or record them.
- Do family history research through an online family history website.

In the Kitchen

Activities can utilize food and beverages with the following suggestions:

- Choose favorite foods and beverages for mealtimes and snacks.
- Dip freshly cut fruit in lemon juice to keep from turning brown.

- Review recipes and reminisce about favorite meals. Sometimes comfort foods remind us of special times and special people and help us feel relaxed and emotionally secure. Utilize these comfort foods for special days.

- Enjoy snacks together. Sometimes when the caregiver eats with your loved one, it allows your loved one to feel relaxed. Smile and communicate gently during the process. Sharing food works as well.

- Make a collage of favorite foods—cut pictures from magazines, and paste them onto construction paper.

- Try a new food or beverage together.

- Take a trip to the grocery store, and read the labels together. Getting out of the house is extremely important.

- Your loved one can participate by helping out in the kitchen with cooking. This can include chopping vegetables or fruit with supervision, spooning cookie dough onto trays, stirring batter, washing fruits or vegetables, draining liquid from canned food, kneading bread dough, peeling hard boiled eggs, greasing cookie sheets, etc.

Trivia/History

Trivia/history is one of the better activities to use with someone who suffers from memory loss. Generally the loss is short-term and despite this, your loved one is able to recall incredible details about the history of the community, family, and country. Some examples:

- Utilize the *How Much Do you Know About* series. There are over 150 different e-Books that give great historical and trivia information on a wide variety of topics available for download at www.TheROSStore.com.

- Most people with memory impairment love to fill in the blank. Utilize old song lines and finish the verse. You can also use old commercial jingles like Burma

Shave and Impala toothpaste. It is easy
to find these by searching online.

- Subscribe to magazines that feature
  information about history like *American
  Heritage* or *Reminisce*. Both magazines
  look at history rather than current events.

- Take walking tours of the downtown
  area wherever you live, and reminisce
  about historical moments in the town.
  It is always good for the caregiver to
  do a little research first to assist along
  the way.

- Talk about historical events from your
  loved one's lifetime and what their
  thoughts were when the events occurred.

Reminiscing

Reminiscing is a quiet, reassuring activity that
draws upon your loved one's earlier life
interests, natural abilities, and skills. These
activities provide opportunities for positive

feelings of self-worth and the value of life
is reaffirmed. Suggested ideas:

- Browse through a box of personal
  keepsakes, such as jewelry, photos,
  fishing items, stamps, coins, patches, etc.
- Have your loved one describe their
  profession or lifetime work.
- Listen to favorite music on the
  appropriate device. If your loved one has
  an old record player, use it.
- Leaf through favorite recipe books.
- Look through school yearbooks. Read
  the autographs.
- Rediscover items in a cedar chest or
  old trunk.
- Share stories about sport trophies,
  photos, or other awards hanging
  in the house.
- View home movies, videos, or slides.
- Do an online search of the old
  family home.

Regardless of the activity type you choose to engage your loved one in, you must engage them. Please commit to at least one activity per day—a game or a conversation. Below are additional suggestions for you to use with your loved one. The specifics of how to engage your loved one will be up to you based on your loved one's remaining abilities. Remember, set them up for success.

Art Activities

- Coloring
- Painting
- Dancing

Writing Activities

- Writing a story or poem
- Writing a letter

perseverating on letters

probably NO

Visual Activities

- Watching a movie
- Watching a performance *online*

Listening Activities

- Music
- Storytelling
- Books on tape
- Listening to the radio

Entertainment Activities

- Board games, card games
- Video games
- Crossword puzzles

Craft Activities

- Jewelry making
- Knitting
- Scrapbooking
- Woodworking

Active Activities

- Dancing
- Folding laundry
- Road trips

Activity Tips for Individuals with Mild to Moderate Dementia

Many loved ones have cognitive deficits that are significant enough to impact their day as well as their awareness of their surroundings. By providing activities that reinforce their past, we can increase and improve their social skills which can improve their general interactions with others.

Validating Activities

Validating activities allow us to validate the memories and positive feelings of individuals who are much disoriented.

Reminiscing Activities

Reminiscing activities are designed to help your loved one identify the important contributions he or she has made throughout their lifetime. It is an important part of human development to see oneself as a contributing member of society.

Resocializing Activities

Once your loved one can successfully participate in reminiscing and validating activities, it is time to encourage them, through resocializing activities, to build on those social skills, and begin to expand their connections to the community in which they live. This can be with a neighbor, within the church, or within their community.

Chapter 8

Activities of Daily Living Tips and Suggestions

Unlike leisure activities, the Activities of Daily Living covered in this book are necessary activities that are a part of everyday life. As you work to adjust your loved one's daily routine, here are some practical tips and suggestions to work into the daily routine concerning the basic ADLs.

Bathing

Bathing can be a relaxing, enjoyable experience or a time of confrontation and anger. For individuals that suffer from any form of dementia, bathing/showering can be a traumatic experience. Use a calm approach. Your loved one's "usual" routine is very important. Many attempts and methods may have to be practiced before finding success, relaxation, and a positive experience.

Safety and Preparation

- Water temperature should range from 110-115 degrees Fahrenheit maximum to prevent burning or skin injury.

- Floor of tub needs skid proofing or a rubber mat.

- Place a nonskid rug on the floor outside the tub to prevent slipping.

- Install grab bars around the tub. Always make sure the grab bars are properly and securely installed into the wall studs.

- Do not use bath oils.

NEVER leave your loved one unattended in the bathroom.

Bathing—Know Your Loved One

- Is your loved one accustomed to a bath or shower?

- Can they get into a bath or shower without assistance?

- If they need help, who is your loved one the most comfortable with when needing assistance bathing?

Bathing—Communicating and Motivating

- Don't ask if they want to bathe. Simply say in an easy, friendly voice, "Bath time."

- Use short, simple sentences.

- Look directly at your loved one.

- One step at a time, follow their normal routine. Wash hair first and then wash body, or soak for 10 minutes before washing. When they finish one step, go to the next.

- Be mindful of the little details— preparation and execution.

- Always smile, talk calmly and gently.

- Do not argue, or try to explain "why."

- If your loved one becomes angry or combative about bathing, **STOP**, and try another time.

Bathing—Customary Routines and Preferences

- How often does your loved one bathe?

- What time of day does your loved one normally bathe? *after breakfast*

- Be sure to have your loved one's favorite personal care products for familiar smell and feeling. *H&S Shampoo*

Bathing—Planning and Executing

- Consider the process that works for the caregiver and loved one when it is time to bathe.

  For example, your loved one needs assistance undressing and getting into the tub. They always remove their shirt first, followed by their pants, socks, and

Sponge bath

underwear. The tub has a built-in seat that is covered with ceramic tile. Your loved one needs a towel laid on the tile prior to sitting down because the tile is cold against their skin. Once seated, your loved one also likes a towel draped over their shoulders so they feel less exposed with you assisting them while they bathe.

- Have all care items and tools ready prior to starting the bath process.

- Have a shower chair if necessary.

- Have a handheld hose for showering and bathing.

- Have a long-handled sponge or scrubbing brush if they would like to scrub themselves.

- Have sponges with soap inside or a soft soap applicator instead of bar soap. Bar soap can easily slip out of your loved one's hand.

- Take one step at a time. When they finish one step, go to the next.

- Remember to **STOP**, and try another time if your loved one becomes angry or combative.

- Use a towel to put over shoulders or on lap so they feel less exposed.

- Have towel and clothing prepared for when the bath is finished.

- Use a terry cloth robe instead of a towel to dry off.

Other Bathroom & Grooming Activities

Brushing Teeth

3 - 2022

Can do on own

- Give them step-by-step directions. This may not be as simple as you think. Take a moment and think of all of the steps necessary to brush your teeth, from walking into the bathroom, to finding the toothpaste in the drawer and removing the cap, to rinsing their mouth once they have finished brushing. Depending on your loved one's level of dementia, it might be easier to show them.

- For family members at home, brush your teeth at the same time.

- Use positive reinforcement, and compliment your loved one on the good job they are doing.

- Help your loved one to clean their dentures as needed.

Trim beard & mustache

Shaving

- Encourage a male to shave.

- Use an electric razor for safety.

- If they need assistance, please provide it.

- Give positive feedback, and do not verbally correct.

For example, if your loved one only managed to shave half of his face, do not criticize and tell him he "did it wrong." Instead, ask if he would like some help.

Makeup

- If your loved one had been accustomed to wearing makeup, there is no reason for this to stop. If she shows interest or desire to wear makeup, encourage her to do so, and offer assistance to apply if needed.

Hair

- Try to maintain hairstyle and care as your loved one did.

- Explain each step simply beforehand to reduce any anxiety.

- When washing hair use nonstinging shampoo.

- Use warm water for washing and rinsing. Give your loved one warning so they will be prepared before you rinse their hair.

Nails

- Keep nails clean and trimmed. Be gentle while trimming your loved one's nails. Be mindful of how you pull and where you place their fingers and arms.

  *NOTE: It is equally important that caregivers maintain clean, short-trimmed fingernails for safety when providing hands-on care with loved ones.

- If your loved one had a normal/weekly schedule for nail care prior to the onset of vascular dementia, please try to maintain that schedule.

- Offer to polish your loved one's nails.

- When polishing, engage your loved one in conversation.

Podiatry for toes.

Toileting or Using the Bathroom

- Mark the bathroom door so it can be identified.

- Learn your loved one's individual habits and routines for using the toilet. This may not be something that you know and is part of the changing roles.

- Toilet routinely on rising, before and after meals, and at bedtime, at minimum.

- If your loved one is having trouble communicating, please watch for agitation, pulling at their clothes, or walking/pacing restlessly. This may be an indication that they need to go to the bathroom.

- Assist with clothing as needed, and be positive and pleasant while assisting.

- Provide verbal cues and instructions as needed, while being guiding, but not controlling.

Clothing

Clothing—Know Your Loved One

- Initially, daily clothing choices should remain as they had been and based on your loved one's available wardrobe.

- As their dementia progresses, changes will have to be made. Clothes need to be comfortable and easy to remove, especially to go to bathroom.

Clothing—Routines and Preferences

- Have a friendly discussion each evening about the next day's schedule and what your loved one may want to wear.

- Remember that as their dementia progresses, changes will have to be made. You may have to limit the choice of clothing, and leave only two outfits in their room at a time.

Have rotation on cardigans

- If your loved one wants to wear the same thing every day, and if you can afford it, buy three or four sets of the same clothing.

- Try to maintain your loved one's preferred dressing routine by laying the clothes out in order of what your loved one prefers to put on first.

Clothing—Planning and Executing

- Choose clothes that are loose fitting and have elastic waistbands.

- Choose wraparound clothing instead of the pullover type.

- You may consider clothing that opens and closes in the front—not the back—for your loved one. This may be helpful in allowing them to dress themselves and maintain some independence

- Choose clothing with large, flat buttons, zippers, or Velcro closures.

- If possible, attach a zipper pull to the end of the zipper to make it easier to zip pants or jackets.

- Choose slip-on shoes, and purchase elastic shoelaces that allow shoes to slip on and off without untying the shoelaces.

Dressing

Dressing—Know Your Loved One

Initially, your loved one may just need verbal cues and instructions on dressing. As their dementia progresses, you will have to take a more active role. Please remember to allow your loved one to dress themselves as long as possible so they can maintain a sense of dignity and independence. You will have to be *Now* the judge of when all caregivers need to begin assisting in the dressing process.

Similar to bathing, you need to identify who your loved one is the most comfortable with when needing care. Female/male, a specific caregiver?

Sex and age of the caregiver can be a significant issue.

Dressing—Communicating and Motivating

- Use short, simple sentences.

- Provide verbal cues and instructions as needed.

- Ask if your loved one would like to go to the toilet before getting dressed.

- If they are confused, give instructions in very short steps, such as, "Now put your arm through the sleeve." It may help to use actions to demonstrate these instructions.

- Give praise as justified for accomplishing each step.

- Always smile, talk calmly and gently.

- Do not argue, or try to explain "why."

- Be guiding, not controlling.

Dressing—Routines and Preferences

- Does your loved one get dressed first thing in the morning—before breakfast or after breakfast?

- Does your loved one change into pajamas right before bed or after dinner?

  ordinarily

- Try to maintain your loved one's preferred routine. For example, they may like to put on all of their underwear before putting on anything else.

Dressing—Planning and Executing

concern at toileting

- Think about privacy—make sure that blinds or curtains are closed and that no one will walk in and disturb your loved one while they are dressing.

- Make sure the room is warm enough to get dressed in.

- Before handing your loved one their clothes, make sure that items are not inside out and that buttons, zips, and fasteners are all undone.

- Hand your loved one only one item at a time.

- If needed, let your loved one get dressed while sitting in a chair that has armrests. This will help your loved one keep their balance.

yes

DRESSING NOTE 1: If mistakes are made—for example, something is put on the wrong way—be tactful, or find a way for you both to laugh about it.

DRESSING NOTE 2: It can be useful if your loved one wears several layers of thin clothing rather than one thick layer, as they can then remove a layer if they feel too warm.

DRESSING NOTE 3: Remember that your loved one may no longer be able to tell you if they are too hot or cold, so keep an eye out for signs of discomfort.

Meals

General Information

- Limit distractions. Serve meals in quiet surroundings, away from the television and other activities.

- Your loved one might not be able to tell if something is too hot to eat or drink. Always test the temperature of foods and beverages before serving.

- Keep long-standing personal preferences in mind when preparing food. However, be aware that your loved one may suddenly develop new food preferences or reject foods that they enjoyed in the past.

- Give your loved one plenty of time to eat. It may take an hour or longer to finish a snack or meal so factor that into the overall schedule for the day.

- Make meals an enjoyable social event so everyone looks forward to the experience.

Eating

Eating—Know Your Loved One

[handwritten: Competence v performance]

- Can your loved one feed themselves?

- Does your loved one have a visual impairment that may affect their ability to see their meal or drink?

  *NOTE: Older individuals tend to perceive bright, deep colors as lighter. They are able to see yellow, orange, and red more easily than darker colors. Due to change in our eyesight as we age, eating and dining offer additional challenges. *[handwritten: ✗]*

Eating—Communicating and Motivating

- Use short, simple sentences.

- Provide verbal cues and instructions as needed.

- Give your loved one your full attention.

- Always smile, talk calmly and gently.

- Do not argue, or try to explain "why."

Eating—Routines and Preferences

- No matter what time of day they eat breakfast, lunch, and dinner, be consistent every day.

- Offer snacks throughout the day.

- Do they eat their meals at the kitchen table? DR only

Eating—Planning and Execution

Eating a meal can be a challenge for your loved one with dementia. There are several areas that need to be taken into account, such as visual impairment, physical ailment, changes in preferences, and dietary restrictions. Here are some simple techniques that can help reduce mealtime problems:

Meal Preparation for Mild Dementia

- If your loved one wants to assist in making a meal:

- o Make sure your cabinets are organized with each item labeled with large easy-to-see labels.

- o Use simple step-by-step written or verbal instructions.

- o You or another caregiver should perform tasks using sharp objects, such as knives, or operation of the stove or oven.

- o When using a stove top, use the back burners, and turn the pot handles inward toward the back of the stove to avoid any potential grabbing of the pots or pans.

- If you are not there to supervise because you have to go to work:

  - o Avoid planning meals that require use of the stove. Your loved one may not remember to turn off the stove and may not be able to distinguish between a pot that is hot or cold.

○ Lay out the ingredients of a meal on the counter or in the refrigerator in labeled containers in the order that your loved one will use them (similar to laying out their clothes at night).

○ Transfer bulk items, including milk, from a larger container to a smaller container that is easier to lift and pour.

Meal Preparation for Higher Level Dementia

- Try to have all meals eaten at a kitchen or dining table, or in a chair with a serving tray. Avoid meals in bed, if possible. Let the bed be for sleeping.

Appropriate Lighting and Eyesight

Chair against Wall?

- Reduce glare by having your loved one sit with the sunlight behind them when eating.

- Use lighting which illuminates the entire dining space and makes objects visible, as well as reducing shadows or reflections.

- Adjust lighting above the table to help see as much detail as possible.

- Remember that older individuals tend to perceive bright, deep colors as lighter. They are able to see yellow, orange, and red more easily than darker colors.

Setting the Table and Serving

- Set each place setting in the same way for every meal. Set it the way your loved one used to. Offer your loved one the opportunity to assist in setting the table.

- Decide how to set the rest of the table— main dish, side dishes, seasonings, and condiments. Do it the same way each day.

- When pouring a light-colored drink, such as milk, use a dark glass.

- When pouring a dark-colored drink, such as cola, use a white glass.

- Avoid clear glasses. They can disappear from view.

meals are composed of a variety of colors

- Use white dishes when eating dark-colored food, and use dark dishes when eating light-colored food.

- To make dishes easier to find on the table, use a tablecloth or placemats that are the opposite color of the dishes.

interesting

- Fiesta wear colors (yellow/tangerine) contrast with most foods so they can be easily seen and will enhance visual perception.

- There should be a clear visual distinction between the table, the dishes, and the food.

- Use solid colors with no distracting patterns.

Chapter 9

Home Preparation

Home preparation is an important part of caregiving. The following are general tips that caregivers and family members can use to prepare the home for your loved one.

General Organization and Environment

It is important to remember your loved one's thought process, and how organization is affected.

When organizing your loved one's environment, if you can, do it *with* them. What works for you, might not work for your loved one.

- Assign everything to a place in the home.

- Always put items back in their place after using them in order to avoid clutter.

- o You may want to go one step further and label drawers and other areas used by your loved one.

- If your loved one has developed problems with motor skills, e.g., walking and balance:

  - o Have your loved one evaluated for the use of a walker or cane.

  - o Remove objects left on the floor, such as shoes, bags, and boxes. These items should be placed in their designated areas of the home. If left out, they can be a tripping hazard.

  - o Keep walkways open and wide.

  - o Use extension cords sparingly, and always secure them out of the places where people walk. Bundle all the cords, and secure them to the wall instead of the floor.

- Remove and avoid clutter on desks, tables, and countertops, and in cabinets and closets. This makes it easier to locate and reach specific items. Your loved one will be less frustrated.

- Install handrails where possible for easier independent movement from one room to the next.

- Leave doors fully opened or closed. Make sure the doors open easily and smoothly and that doorknobs are securely fastened to the door, especially if your loved one has tremors.

- Remove throw rugs. If you must use them, *done* opt for slide-resistant rugs that can be taped or tacked down.

- Identify and address flooring issues. Check every floor, walkway, threshold, and entry. Remove or fix loose floorboards, uneven tiles, loose nails, or carpeting that has bunched up over time.

Furniture

- Make sure there is enough room to move around. If possible, place furniture pieces 5½ feet from each other so your loved one can move comfortably around the room, especially if they are in a wheelchair.

- Use chairs with straight backs, armrests, and firm seats. Where possible, add firm cushions to existing pieces to add height. This will make it easier for your loved one to get up and sit down.

Lighting

Depending on your loved one's eye condition, symptoms from vascular dementia, or individual preference, the need for additional or less lighting could be key in their safety and ability to perform tasks independently.

- If possible, purchase touch lamps or those that can be turned on or off by sound.

- Be certain that all stairwells are well lit and have handrails.

Wandering and Leaving Home without Supervision

You may encounter your loved one attempting to leave to go out for a walk, or believing they need to be somewhere. You may want to install some type of system that will alert you when doors are opened and your loved one may be attempting to leave.

yes

Chapter 10

Put Your Mask on First

There will be many challenges to you personally in this caregiving journey that can and will wear you down. As a caregiver, first and foremost, you must take care of yourself in order to be able to assist your loved one. That might be easier said than done, but please make every effort to do so. The following are some general tips for you, the family caregiver:

About You

- Put yourself first (this is not being selfish); if you are not in good physical or mental health you cannot help anyone.

- Arrange some time for yourself.

- Keep a strong support system.

- Do not be afraid to ask for help.

- Keep contact with friends.

- Define priorities; do not try to be all things to all people.

Stress

- Recognize your own stress, and take steps to minimize. Stress can be exhibited in multiple ways:
  - Anger
  - Helplessness
  - Embarrassment
  - Grief
  - Depression
  - Isolation
  - Physical illness

Burnout

Burnout for caregivers results from physical and emotional exhaustion.

It is important to realize a family member, spouse, or hired caregiver experiences the same emotions as staff in health care facilities, but may not have the needed support system. Suggestions to avoid burnout:

- Know what makes you angry or impatient. Make a list.

- Look for the reason behind behavior.

- Use relaxation techniques, e.g., deep breathing, imagery, and music.

- Ask for help, and accept help when it is offered!

Caregiving is a challenging road with constant twists and turns, from the change in your role/relationship with your loved one, to dealing with the strains of a 24/7 job of caring for that loved one. As much as you may feel like you are alone, please know that you are not. Millions of family caregivers are dealing with the same issues that you are. Do not be embarrassed to share details about what you are experiencing, and do not be afraid to ask for help. There are individuals, organizations, and support groups throughout the country

that are available to you. There is also R.O.S.—
built on the simple mission of our founder's
need to help his mother and father during a
25-year battle with Parkinson's and dementia.
We understand what you are going through,
and we are here to help.

Personal History Form

This is _____'s Personal History

Name: _____

Maiden Name: _____

Date of Birth: _____

Preferred Name: _____

Name and relationship of people completing this history:

_____

_____

_____

What age do you think the person thinks they are?

_____

Do they ask for their spouse/partner but do not recognize them?

_____

Do they look for their children but do not recognize them?

_____

Do they look for their mom? _____

Do they perceive themselves as younger? Please describe.

_____

_____

Describe the "home" they remember. _____

_____

_____

_____

Describe the person's personality prior to the onset of

dementia. _____

_____

_____

What makes the person feel valued? Talents, occupation,

accomplishments, family, etc. _____

_____

_____

What are some favorite items they must always have in

sight or close by? _____

_____

_____

What is their exact morning routine?

_____

_____

_____

_____

What is their exact evening routine?

_____

_____

_____

_____

What type of clothing do they prefer? Do they like to choose their own clothes for the day, or do they prefer to have their clothes laid out for them?

_____

_____

_____

_____

What is their favorite beverage?

_____

What is their favorite food?

_____

What will get them motivated? (Church, friends coming over, going out, etc.)

_____

_____

_____

_____

List significant interests in their life, such as hobbies, recreational activities, job related skills/experiences, military experience, etc.

- Age 8 to 20:

_____

_____

_____

- Age 20 to 40:

_____

_____

_____

What is their religious background? (Affiliation, prayer time, symbols, traditions, church/synagogue name, etc. Did they lead any services or sing in the choir?)

_____

_____

_____

What type of music do they enjoy listening to, playing, or singing? Do they have any musical talents?

_____

_____

_____

What is their favorite TV program? Movie?

_____

_____

_____

Did they enjoy reading? Which authors, topics, or genres do they prefer? Would they listen to audiobooks or books on tape?

_____

_____

_____

_____

Can they tell the difference between someone on TV and a real person?

_____

_____

Include names of spouses/partners, dates of marriage, and other relevant information. (If married more than once, provide specifics for each partner.)

_____

_____

_____

_____

_____

List distinct characteristics about his/her
spouse/partner(s), such as occupations, personality traits,
or daily routine.

_____

_____

_____

_____

_____

Do they have children? Be sure to include children both
living and deceased. Include names, birth dates, and any
other relevant information.

_____

_____

_____

_____

_____

Who do they ask for the most? What is their relationship
with this person(s)? Describe how that person typically
spends their day.

_____

_____

_____

_____

What causes your loved one stress?

_____

_____

_____

_____

What calms them down when they are stressed or agitated?

_____

_____

_____

_____

Other information that would help bring joy to your loved one.

_____

_____

_____

_____

_____

_____

_____

_____

_____

About the Authors

Scott Silknitter

Scott Silknitter is the founder of R.O.S. Therapy Systems. He designed and created the R.O.S. Play Therapy™ System, the *How Much Do You Know About* Series of themed activity books and the R.O.S. *BIG Book*. Starting with a simple backyard project to help his mother and father, Scott has dedicated his life to improving the quality of life for all seniors through meaningful education, entertainment, and activities.

Robert D. Brennan, RN, NHA, MS, CDP

Robert Brennan is a Registered Nurse and Nursing Home Administrator with over 35 years of experience in long-term care. He is a Certified Dementia Practitioner and is Credentialed in Montessori-Based Dementia Programming (MBDP) providing general and Train the Trainer programs. Robert was responsible for the development of an Assisted Living Federation of America (ALFA) "Best of the Best" award-winning program for care of individuals with dementia using MBDP. He currently provides education on dementia and long-term regulatory topics.

Alisa Tagg, BA, ACC/EDU, AC-BC, CDP

Alisa Tagg is a Certified Activity Consultant with a specialization in Education and a Certified Dementia Practitioner. With over 20 years of industry experience, Alisa is an authorized certification instructor for the Modular Education Program for Activity Professionals. Alisa currently serves as the President of the National Association of Activity Professionals.

References

1. *The Handbook of Theories on Aging* (Bengtson et al., 2009)
2. *Activity Keeps Me Going, Volume 1* (Peckham et al., 2011)
3. *Essentials for the Activity Professional in Long-Term Care* (Lanza, 1997)
4. *Abnormal Psychology*, Butcher
5. www.dhspecialservices.com
6. National Certification Council for Dementia Practitioners www.NCCDP.org
7. "Managing Difficult Dementia Behaviors: An A-B-C Approach" By Carrie Steckl
8. Iowa Geriatric Education Center website, Marianne Smith, PhD, ARNP, BC Assistant Professor University of Iowa College of Nursing
9. *Excerpts taken from "Behavior...Whose Problem is it?" Hommel, 2012
10. *Merriam-Webster's Dictionary*
11. "The Latent Kin Matrix" (Riley, 1983)
12. *Care Planning Cookbook* (Nolta et al.2007)
13. "Long-Term Care" (Blasko et al. 2011)
14. "Success Oriented Programs for the Dementia Client" (Worsley et al 2005)
15. Heerema, Esther. "Eight Reasons Why Meaningful Activities Are Important for People with Dementia." www.about.com
16. *Validation: The Feil Method* (Feil, 1992)
17. *Activities 101 for the Family Caregiver* (Appler-Worsley, Bradshaw, Silknitter)
18. American Foundation for the Blind
19. www.aging.com
20. www.WebMD.com
21. www.ninds.nih.gov
22. www.caregiver.org
23. www.alz.org

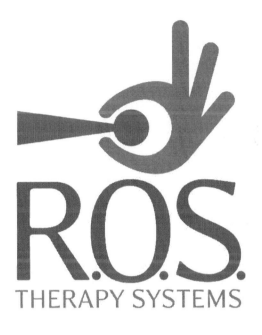

R.O.S.
THERAPY SYSTEMS

For additional assistance, please contact us at:
www.ROSTherapySystems.com
888-352-9788

Made in the USA
Columbia, SC
17 February 2022

56400119R00063